CHASING THE TALE

CHASING THE TALE:

Thoughts from a Professional Husband

By

Broderick X. Thomas

Copyright © 2007 Broderick Thomas
All rights reserved

ISBN: 978-0-557-03493-2

Third Edition

Publisher:
Atlex Publishing
P.O. Box 3128
Richmond, VA 23228

Published:
November 15, 2011

Cover Design:
Grafxguild

For More Information:
www.theprofessionalhusband.com

Dedication

I dedicate this book to my mother,
Rose Thomas, and my father,
Prince Thomas, Sr. (both deceased)…
without them this would not have been possible.

They made me; they molded me; they matured me.
Although they could not give me perfection,
they gave me the best of them!

Acknowledgements

I would first like to acknowledge some specific women who, at some point in time, have occupied my life and my heart: (in alphabetical order) Cherie, Margaret, Tamara, Tina, Tracey, and Tracie. Without the experiences that I shared with these women, there would be no book.

I would also like to thank the ladies in my family who gave me a ton of support while I was completing this project: my sisters, Dwanda and Tabytha; my sister-in-law, Cylvia; and my niece, Chandra.

Finally, I want to mention a few friends:
Tanisha and Tanisha (pronounced differently) –
two very special women who are continuously challenging me to be better! And K.

Table of Contents

i.	Introduction	15
I.	Self Understanding	21
II.	Love	29
III.	Communication	37
IV.	Togetherness	45
V.	Romance	53
VI.	Respect	61
VII.	Trust	69
VIII.	Commitment	77
IX.	Finances	83
X.	Final Thoughts	91
xi.	Afterword	99

Introduction

My wonderful mother was always a god-fearing woman and she brought me up as a child in a small Episcopal church in Southern Virginia. Now if you've never been to an Episcopal Church service, then I need to explain to you first that it's nothing like a Baptist or Holiness service with hand-clappin', finger-poppin' choirs and the loud-shoutin', Holy Ghost givin' preachers. No, no, no – this is a very calm and monotone service with soothing hymnals and a structured program that you follow along with in a book that is provided for you in the pews. This book is called "The Book of Common Prayer" and in it is the text for every Episcopal service there is – from regular Sunday church services to baptisms to funerals – and even wedding services. Aaahh! Herein lies the reason I've been sharing my childhood churchgoing experience with you because it was in these quiet Sunday morning services that I would ignore the preacher's sermon and turn to the "Order of Holy Matrimony" in the *Book of Common Prayer*. I would daydream about how my first wedding would be and as I read through the service I would insert the name of whichever young girl was holding my attention at the time. I would envision this young lady (who probably was in no way having these same thoughts about me on that particular morning) in her luxurious white gown and me standing with her in front of Father Whatshisname (who was now in full stride with his sermon), and all of our family and friends were out in the congregation sharing this special day with us. He turns and asks me, "Do you, Broderick take this woman…" and I quickly respond, "I do." And then he repeats to her, "Do you, *(insert name here)*, take this man…" She looks up into my eyes with the most endearing smile and answers, "I do." And as the preacher continues, "By the power vested in me, I now pronounce you man and wife…", I realize that in real life he is winding down towards the end of his sermon. So I pause the remainder of the fantasy – which covers the wedding reception, the honeymoon, and the birth of our first child – so that I can stand up and mouth the words to the hymnal that is about to soon follow. In the back of my mind, I'm thinking that I can pick this fantasy up at next week's service; although I'm fully aware that by then the bride in this script will probably have changed at least once. But it was this daydreaming that got me through those Sunday morning services (which, by the way, allowed me pick up a little spirituality) and it was there that the "fairy" tale began…and I've been chasing it ever since.

Now I know that when you first heard the name of this book, "Chasing The Tale", that you probably thought that I was some sort of perverted, wanna-be-player who was out to make a quick buck by telling people about his exploits of the female species. But mind the spelling. Chasing the "t-a-i-l" would have referred to the masculine hunt of the sexual pleasures that women have to offer us. And don't get me wrong, I'm no saint and thereby guilty of doing that too. But the "t-a-l-e" that I wanna talk about is the fairy tale that I shared with you when I began this story. It's not about big booties and erotic escapades, but about connections of two souls and lifelong passions. It is **this** tale that I've been chasing that has brought me to a point of in my life in which I can now accurately refer to myself as "the professional husband". I am permitted to have this title because I have been married **and** divorced three times (yep, you read that right - THREE times) to three different women. In addition to the three marriages, I have also been engaged on three other separate occasions.

The word "engaged" meaning that there have been three instances where I have bought a woman a ring, asked that particular woman to marry me, and her answer was "yes".

And although this may seem like an entire lifetime's worth of romance, all of this has come to pass prior to me obtaining the ripe, yet tender age of 30. Now. The ironic part to this is that I am helplessly willing to take the sacred nuptials again. And no - it's not because I am trying to see how high I can run up my tally on ex-wives. I genuinely believe in the concepts of love, marriage, and family. I'm quite certain that this is because I remember my childhood being centered within a happy household. Some of my earliest memories are of my mom and dad hosting family gatherings at our house. There was always food and drinks and my parents and their friends would laugh and joke and sit around playing cards. I would always wait until my dad had tossed down a few beers so that while he was playing cards, I could convince him to let me have a sip of one (which my mother never liked). But everybody always seemed to have a good time and in my eyes, my parents were these popular icons that people just naturally wanted to be around! And I felt as though I was a part of that. I also remember them getting all dressed up to go out to dances and/or parties (especially on New Year's Eve) and we would take pictures of them before they left the house. You just **had** to take pictures because every year it was something to see. My mom loved to sew and she would make herself these drop-dead gorgeous dresses that she complimented with diamond broaches, matching sashes, and a church hat that she wore cocked to one side. She was absolutely exquisite! But not to be outdone, my father would make his entrance having donned the finest of suits (which perfectly complimented my mother's attire) with a really classy tie or bowtie and matching handkerchief, patent leather shoes, and yes – he topped it off with a derby hat of his own from his collection. They seemed to be the ideal couple and every time I saw them in those scenarios, they always looked like they were so in love and the best of friends. And it was these moments – these memories – that forged an everlasting image in my brain as to what love and marriage was supposed to look and feel like. Now, I know that they had their problems like everyone else, but the point is that they never let me see them; and they were married for over thirty years – right up until the death of my father. So that left me to spend my entire adolescence and early adulthood searching for that "forever" type relationship that I grew up around; hence, the tale I've been chasing. I must point out that I have a brother and two sisters who grew up in the same family environment as I did, and each of them have only been married to one person in their whole life! But not me...I'm the one who had to prove Darwin's "trial-by-error" theory when it comes to marriage.

Is that the right guy who made that theory?

But although I've had a few unsuccessful attempts at **keeping** "the knot" tied, I cannot bring myself to relinquish the idea that I **can** get this right. I can have a happy, fulfilling, and yes, a lasting marriage! I know I can. And the reason that I'm so convinced of this is that while I have had quite a few "better halves", I have learned something from them all. Each and every one of them (in their own special way) has taught me valuable lessons about women and what it is that they want and require. Mind you though, these lessons have not come without costs. I'll grant you that some of this education has been fun and enjoyable; but, a large part of it has been tedious, expensive, and all too painful! But you know what? I'm still standing; and I think that's saying something. And because of that, I have chosen to utilize my marriage-filled history to try to offer what may only be the smallest amount of help to others who are in, or about to be in, a relationship of any significance. It is my hope that the men who read this book might take heed to some of my opinions and spare themselves from some of the many mistakes I've made; and that the women who choose to indulge me in my attempt to be a writer will, in fact, pick up a few insights as to how men think and why we think that way.

Please keep in mind ladies, I am in no way trying to pass my thoughts and actions off as those of every man in the world...but I do happen to think of myself as a typical guy, so my opinions may give you a basic starting point.

So, from my many experiences in the marital universe, I would like to now share with you in the subsequent pages of this book my most profound opinions, beliefs, and realizations regarding what I feel are the key components of any and every relationship. These are the thoughts of a professional husband.

I: Self-Understanding

I chose this subject as my starting point because it was the one thing that I didn't (nor couldn't) learn from any of my female counterparts, or anyone else for that matter…it was something I had to figure out on my own. And essentially, that's exactly what self-understanding is – learning yourself, for yourself, all by yourself.

Now ladies, I want you to know that this chapter will primarily relate to the male perspective because hey, that's all I know. But please read on because this is some of that insight that I thought you would enjoy…

Now, "all by yourself" can be a hard concept for someone like me because part of the reason that I've been in and out of so many relationships is that for the largest portion of my adult life, I <u>was afraid to be alone</u>. In fact, as of the time I began writing this book, it has only been a few months since I got up the nerve and took the opportunity to live by myself for the very first time in my life.

I know, I've been a big baby all this time! But follow along – you'll see that I've been working on it!

I think I mentioned before that I grew up in a small town in southern Virginia in my parent's home. And like most small town teenagers, I could not wait to graduate high school and go off to some big city to claim my freedom as an adult. I had come to the conclusion that the easiest and fastest way for me to begin my worldwide travels would be to join the military; so I enlisted in the U.S. Air Force. That's right, I had a one-way ticket to becoming my own man and Uncle Sam was footing the bill. However, the solitude for which I searched would be put on hold because I found out upon arriving at "boot camp" in San Antonio, Texas that I would be living in a dormitory where there would be fifty of us sharing the same roof. I had just gone from my mother telling me what to do to a drill sergeant telling me what to do; but now it was as if I had forty-nine nagging little brothers to contend with as well. We had to sleep together, shower together; we even had to march in-step together whenever we were outside walking around the base. But I just kept telling myself that this was only for six weeks, and soon I would be on my way to independence and singularity at my next duty station. As it turns out, Uncle Sam wasn't quite as concerned with my quest for isolation as he was with finding the most cost-effective way to train me to do a job for him. So, from Lackland Air Force Base in Texas, I was shipped out to Lowry Air Force Base in Denver, Colorado.

Now, I had been told that in Denver the women outnumbered the men at a ratio of eight-to-one, so at this point I'm thinking that things are starting to take a turn for the better.

Upon my arrival in the Mile High City, I was pleasantly informed that I would be living in yet another dormitory with as many as three hundred other students for the duration of my technical training. Now me being an eighteen year old hot-head, this would normally have been the time when I lost my composure and threw a tantrum because things weren't going my way. But as the old cliché goes, there's a silver lining in every cloud. Apparently the United States Air Force, in their infinite wisdom, had deemed it prudent for young men and women to be able to share sleeping quarters in the same building while they were being trained. It was a CO-ED dormitory!!!! And as you can imagine, the idea of being alone was now being abandoned with more velocity than the supersonic jets that I was there to learn about! To speed the story up a little, it was here that I met and married Wife #1; and the rest, as they say, is history. I somehow got caught up in the idea that I was supposed to be with someone; it was almost as if being alone caused some freakish response in my behavior that I really would rather not endure. From that point on, I've always lived with either a girlfriend/fiancé or a wife or a roommate or a relative…anybody to keep from being alone. Finally, after all of my travels and various cohabitants, I began to realize that there was a problem in my psyche. I had not established within myself who "I" was or who I wanted to become. I was drifting from person to person; each time conforming my identity to accommodate whoever was in my life at that time. If my wife liked being a "homebody", then I liked being one too. If my girlfriend liked being in the club scene, then that's where I wanted to be!

If you've ever seen it, this kinda reminds me of that movie "The Runaway Bride" where Julia Roberts eats whatever style of eggs her current fiancé likes, but in the end she has to find out for herself what style of eggs she actually likes. Anyway...

This critical revelation is what led me to make the commitment to take the time to evaluate myself and come to understand "me", and ultimately mature into the man that you are presently reading about.

Let's talk about that word "man" for a second because it is actually a concept that is very important to my case about men developing self-understanding. Upon taking on the project of evaluating myself, the first thing that I had to accept was that I was not yet a "man" (according to what I knew the word to mean) and this was occurring to me somewhere around the time I was twenty-eight or twenty-nine years old. But I was only able to arrive at this conclusion because I was getting close to the point of being able to bear that title, and I could feel it. At this stage in my life, I could tell that I was starting to mature and think differently about my life; and I was beginning to make responsible decisions and choices like I never had before. It was becoming painfully obvious to me that I had not been doing those things before now (at least not consistently); therefore, I had not been a "man" before now.

I hope that in this conversation you all picked up on the age I just mentioned. The point to that is that every man matures at a different time in his life than other men – some at age twenty, some at age thirty, and some not until even forty or beyond…but every man is different.

Before my father died, he used to have me sit with him on the steps out in front of his business and we would have these deep conversations about life. He taught me early on that being a man has nothing to do with your age, your social status, or any material possessions that you may have acquired. He said that being a man was about taking responsibility for all that was yours!

"If she's **your** wife…you care for her; if they're **your** children…you provide for them; if it's **your** house…you maintain and protect it.", he said to me on one particular occasion.

He went on to state that, as a man, any actions that you take or words that you speak, you must own up to them; in spite of the fact that consequences may exist.

"When you decide you want to live by those rules, then you can call yourself a man and can't nobody question it!" my father finished.

Now although I'd been carrying these words of wisdom from my paternal creator around since the pubescent age of twelve, I was nearly thirty years old before I had the audacity and good sense to actually apply them in my life. And I'm sure that my inability to utilize this wisdom early on has undoubtedly contributed to my unsuccessful attempts at being a good husband or mate. As I reflected back on those early relationships, I had to ask myself; if I didn't know what it meant to be a man, then how could I have known what I was supposed to be doing with a woman? I guess that just means that sometimes the best lessons are the ones that take a while to learn.

Now after all of this "self-evaluation" had taken place and I had begun to realize my rite of passage into manhood, the next task was to identify the **type** of man that I ultimately wanted to become. And this is one of those things that you really want to spend some time thinking about because if you're going to seriously commit to achieving this persona, you want to be fairly certain that it's the right one for you. I actually took the approach of envisioning my funeral and determining the things that I would want to be said about me during my eulogy; and from there, I decided to work my way backwards in figuring out how I could achieve those characteristics. This was tough for me because it meant that in addition to recognizing my strengths and capabilities, I also had to admit my faults and flaws as well. Can you imagine having to confront yourself with issues like: "I guess I'm really not that good with handling money" or "Maybe I'm not as spiritual as I thought I was" and "I do have a problem with seeing things through to the end?" But these were all things that could be corrected over time, and I had just made the first step by confessing them as my shortcomings. So, I began to attend church on a more regular basis than I had been before, and I eventually joined a local branch of Zion. I not only went to regular Sunday services, but I also frequented mid-week Bible Studies and participated in some of the ministries that were available as well. This was important to me because I believe that in order to truly be a man, you must first be a man *of God* because he is the one who created us as such to begin with.

I want to say that I do not profess to be Billy Graham or anybody like that; but I simply want to acknowledge my spiritual relationship with God – which probably is the result of all that daydreaming I did in church as a kid.

As my next order of business, I began to work on becoming more conscious of dealing with my money. I enrolled myself in a program to have my credit restored, I took the time to prepare and document my personal budget, and I even took the initiative to begin investing money for my future savings and retirement. For the record, I'm not quite sure at this particular moment how I'm doing with seeing things through to the end; but if you are reading this book, then that probably means that I have made some progress with that. Now please understand that I'm not telling you all of this in order to brag about anything that I have or have done; I am simply sharing with you how engaging in the exercise of self-understanding played a significant role in bringing me to the more mature level of manhood in which I now exist. And this venture was important for me because I had not received the benefit of learning the concept of manhood from an experienced practitioner. You see, it has occurred to me that the most efficient path to manhood is to have a man around who can train you to be one. Normally, a father (or stepfather) can help instill in us the proper values of being a man and impart that certain wisdom that can help us avoid the pitfalls that have plagued their own lives. They can teach and guide and correct us early on, so that when we are old enough we can look back on those lessons with a new degree of understanding and realize the practical application for the present circumstances. But my father was not available to provide those kinds of things for me for very long - he died just before I turned thirteen years old. So there was a missing element for me during those crucial adolescent years in which a young lad is supposed to be molded into a responsible carrier of the Y-chromosome. And there was to be no stepfather in the picture for our household either, because my mother was one of those "one-man-for-a-lifetime" kinda girls.

I wonder why she couldn't have passed on to me that particular chromosome.

Therefore, I have had to take the non-traditional route to male development through trial and error, and learning from my mistakes; and boy, have there been a lot of mistakes.

*I've often been known to say, "I may not know what to do as a husband, but I definitely know what **not** to do!"*

Those mistakes, especially when it comes to women, are the basis on which this book is written and the catalyst for me learning to understand myself. There just came a point in my life when I started to realize that in all of my failed romances, the one common factor was me, and maybe it was time to do something about it. Undertaking this endeavor has revealed a lot of things to me, though; one of which is how these same concepts can be used to improve relationships between men and women (which I haven't forgotten was our original focus, by the way). Remember how I started out about understanding and evaluating ourselves? Well, I believe we should also understand and evaluate our relationships on a regular basis as well. We should spend the time with our counterpart trying to openly identify the strengths and weaknesses that exist in our relationship and commit to developing reasonable strategies that focus on our fortes and minimize the flaws. For instance, if romance is a strong suit between the two of you, but you have a hard time agreeing on what to watch on television, then spend lots of time at candlelit dinners and romantic getaways; then, either form a rotating schedule for the tube, get a VCR, or invest in TiVo! The next step is to follow all of that up with determining how we ultimately want our relationship to be and take the necessary steps to get there. We should try to imagine how we want our golden years to be and talk about the things that we can do together to achieve that image. You see where I'm going with this now? Good, because as I bear my heart and soul in the remaining pages, it'll all come back to what I've just shared with you. Stick with me…this could get interesting!

II: Love

Ideally, this would have been the first thing that I talked about because love is supposed to be what everything else in a relationship is based on. But in my eyes, I felt that the whole "self-understanding" thing was a prerequisite to anything else I had to say, so I juggled the batting order a little bit.
Now ladies, at this point I would like to apologize to you all for the use of my sports analogies and any other "guy" verbiage you will notice throughout the rest of my scribblings. I would say "It's a just a guy thing", but I'm sure most of you have heard that more than enough, so I'll just leave it at the apology!

With that being said, I have to assume that it is obvious to everyone that love is a given in any serious relationship. Well, then again, we all know what can happen when we **ass-u-me** things; so let me just say this to be sure that everyone understands my position. If you don't love someone, then you should not be with them! Now that I have that off of my chest, there's really only one other point that I want to make about the subject.

We all know that there is a difference between "loving" a person and being "in love" with them.
You did know that, right?
I mean, I "love" my mom and my sisters, but I am not "in-love" with them. I have also experienced being in a relationship and really "loving" someone – and by that I

mean that I deeply cared for them and would do whatever was possible to keep any harm from befalling them – but I did not feel the passion of being "in-love" with them. And I know that that will sound like a typical "guy cop-out" to the ladies, but I believe that there is a reasonable amount of validity to this concept; and it is this validity that allows me to separate the two ideas for individual analyzation and application. For instance, I have come to the conclusion that being "in-love" is a superficial emotion…it's temporary. Wait, wait, wait…let me explain. I think that being "*in* love" is that feeling you get from the excitement of someone new. You know, when you first start dating a person and you get butterflies in your stomach when you're about to see them, or when you just think about that person for a minute and you start smiling for no reason. Next thing you know – "I think I'm in love!" It is, without a doubt, the absolute greatest feeling in the world! And if I had a hundred dollars for every time I've said those words, I'd have more than…well let's not talk numbers, but just know that I've said it more than you might care to imagine. And you know what? Every time I've said it, I've meant it. Honestly; every woman that I have ever proposed to (and quite a few others), I was truly in love with – at that particular time. So what happened? What went wrong? Well let me see if I can explain to you the one part that I didn't really understand until later. Let's say a year or two has gone by since I "fell in love" with a particular woman. All of a sudden, the butterflies aren't showing up anymore. Now, there are no more goofy smiles when I was sitting around all alone thinking about her. What does that mean? It means that the temporary feeling of being "in-love" has diminished – not necessarily gone away, but it's just not as intense as it was at first. Now, here's my brilliant realization. What needed to have happened during all of this time is that my "in-love" was supposed to be replaced by just genuine "love" for this lady. I mean, by now I should truly care for her and have come to respect her…all of those fundamental and more permanent emotions should now exists. But knowing me, by now we were probably living together, paying bills together, or maybe even married…you know, the not-so-extraordinary stuff. The excitement and butterflies of "in-love" are gone forever. Or are they? Remember, I said that "in-love" is a temporary emotion created by the excitement of something new? Well I have found that we can continue to recreate those conditions as many times as we like. As long as the "true love" was there, I and my mate could renew the "in-love" emotion by "spicing things up"…trying something new.

Here's a story. While with my second fiancé (who came between Wife #2 and Wife #3), things had gotten to a point where we were really becoming stagnant in our engagement. It seemed like we were always dealing with serious issues in our relationship, or paying bills, or planning the wedding. And although I know that all of those things are very important anytime two people are involved in a responsible relationship, it still didn't keep me from time to time just feeling "blah". So one week in the spring, when we had a long weekend coming up, I decided to make the drive to pick her up (I was in Virginia and she was in New Jersey) and we took a four-day road trip. We stayed in a different hotel every night (and I always requested that our room have a jacuzzi in it), and covered over a thousand miles in four days. And it wasn't like we went across the country or anything – no, we just kinda wandered between her hometown and mine, going no place in particular. We went sightseeing, had romantic dinners, and spent plenty of time just enjoying conversation during the hours that we were riding in the car. And you know what, by the end of our trip, we were "in love" again! When I took her home on the last day, she told me that I had made love to her mind as well as her body.

Man, you should have seen the "S" on my chest once I heard that! But I digress.

The point is that during those times of normal routines and ordinary lifestyles, we had to do something <u>out</u> of the ordinary to get the "in-love" feeling back. And it doesn't have to be a four-day road trip. It could be visiting the sights and attractions in your own town that neither of you have seen before or meeting each other out one night for a date and pretending that the two of you are strangers having dinner for the first time. For the guys, it may even be something simple like having flowers sent to her at work or giving her a candlelit bubble bath one night with rose pedals sprinkled in her water.

FYI fellas, I've always gotten a <u>really</u> good response from that last one!

And ladies, you can try surprise tickets to his favorite sports/music event or the occasional "evening of pampering" that ultimately ends up in a steamy joint shower and you giving him a back massage before bed.

And girls, remember that when you do the joint shower thing as part of "pampering night", the shower is for him - which means that you only get to hog the hot water <u>after</u> he's finished.

Whatever you chose, just know that every so often you have to do **something** to break the monotony. As I said before, being in love is the greatest feeling in the world, no matter how temporary it may be. And because it is, I have been trying to recreate that feeling as many times as humanly possible.

Now the trick for me is to learn to recreate the feeling numerous times, but just with a single person for an extended period.

Remember, the true "love" should take care of itself because that's what love is...it's permanent, it's serious, and it's pure. It is the feeling of knowing that the person that you have chosen to spend your life with is your earth...your world. When I say that, I mean that true love is the genuine feeling that you are grounded in another person...that you exist as a part of them, and they as a part of you. I personally believe that it is that type of true love that comes only from God because just as we cannot control who we love; neither can we control God – it is he who controls us. And his type of love is unconditional, just as ours should be. I've always felt that unconditional love for someone is the kind where we never have any reasons why we feel that way. Whenever I have been asked by my significant other, "Why do you love me?"; if I truly loved that person, then my answer would be, "Just because." Now I know that sounds like a cop-out and as if I were just trying to get out of having a meaningful conversation. But in fact it was quite the opposite. I would intentionally give that answer so that I could go on to explain my belief that if a person can tell you, " I love you because you make me laugh" or "I love you because you take good care of me"; then it is in fact a "conditional" love. I mean, what happens if we stop making them laugh or we can no longer take care of them? Does the love then stop because those conditions don't exist anymore? I don't think that's the way it's supposed to work. If so, I don't believe it's **true** and **unconditional** love because I honestly cannot explain to you why I felt the way that I did about any woman that I have ever truly loved. Granted, I probably should not have loved some of them anyway, but I couldn't help it and I can't explain why I did. It was just because.

Now gentlemen, whenever I've used the "just because" answer, I really and truly meant it. If you should decide to use it (along with the explanation) as a come-on line, please first check to be sure that the lady you are saying it to has not read this book. It won't be a happy ending for you if she has heard it from me first!

Now, I think the reason for the blissful ignorance is because love is one of those inexplicable emotions that comes from the deepest thresholds of who we are. To try to describe what I mean, I want to go back to a movie that came out a few years ago called "The Wedding Crashers".

In case you haven't noticed yet, I am a movie buff...therefore I will from time to time refer to a movie of my liking to illustrate some of my noble thoughts.

In this movie, there is a part that captures the essence of everything that I believe true love to be - in one line. It is the scene where one of the main characters first introduces himself to the girl he has targeted as his prey for the last wedding of the season, which happens to be her sister's wedding. As they are talking, he says to her, "I believe that true love is the soul's recognition of its counterpoint in another." Now I don't know if that came from some poet or from one of the movie's writers, but I thought the statement itself was absolute brilliance! I mean, think about it, we all want to be able to share our lives with someone who shares the same values, beliefs, and dreams as we do, but is still just enough of an opposite to compliment all of the things that we lack. It is something that you don't have to put any effort into; it is just there, and both of your souls can recognize it in the other. You never have to think about it and there is never any reason for it; it is just the presence of caring that two people share in the deepest levels of their existence. I desperately believe that it is that kind of interconnection that allows two people to love each other through eternity.

Now on the other hand, the "in-love" is a totally different story. This, I believe, is the ultimate effect of a chemical balance that is centered on our unique personal choices and preferences.
Which is maybe why they call it "chemistry"?
You see, we all harbor a domineering response to the things that we like and the things that look and feel good to us. And when there is a creature that triggers those reactions in our inner being, it sets off something within our essence that feeds on our strongest emotions of desire. It causes us to temporarily lose control of our reasonable senses, which leads us to do crazy things and act crazy ways.
Lord knows, I have done some craaazy things; but I would need another whole book to tell you about <u>all</u> of them!
But it is this same craziness that makes this feeling of being "in love" so desirable to each and every one of us. It this craziness that drives us to continue to seek out this feeling, no matter how hurtful the last encounter with it may have been. But it is good; it is beautiful; and as I've said numerous times before, it is the most wonderful feeling in the world. Mind you, <u>falling</u> in love is rather easy; it's the <u>staying</u> in love that takes some work. But I promise you all, that no matter how much work it takes, it is worth it because being "in-love" with the person you love (and who also loves you) is one of the greatest joys of life. Who would know that better than me? "Mr. In-Love" himself!

35

III: Communication

"Honey, let's sit down and talk", she says.
"Talk? About what?" he replies.
"Oh nothing in particular; whatever comes to mind. I just think we should spend some time talking."

And there it is. Nine times out of ten, every one of us (whether male or female) has been on one side or the other of that particular conversation. It actually brings to mind the image of a fisherman that throws his line out, hooks the big one and starts reeling the fish in while he's flopping and splashing in resistance all the way.
From a guy's perspective, that is.
Now, bear with me through this part because although I may start to ramble a little bit, I want to be sure you take my point that communication is one of, if not **the** most important elements of a relationship. I'll start off with a story.

One of my closest friends, a man who is twenty-five years my senior and has become my mentor in recent years, would always tell me that his wife had thirty thousand words per day that she <u>had</u> to use. He would say that they were kind of like vacation hours that you accumulate throughout the year at your job…you either have to use 'em or you lose 'em. And since she would only get to exert about fifteen thousand of those words during the course of her workday, the remaining fifteen thousand were left for him alone to absorb at home. Now while this analogy may seem rather extreme (as well as quite comical), I have found the concept of what he was telling me to be somewhat true. Let's be honest, women enjoy being able to talk to someone – it's almost as if it is a form of relaxation.

Ladies, I mean no disrespect; I'm simply stating the facts as I know them. Please try to remember that you have enjoyed my work up to this point…

Furthermore, if there were a utopian society, every woman would be happiest when the person that she spent at least ninety percent of her time talking to was the man who held her affection. Men, on the other hand, don't like to use a lot of unnecessary words – we get a question, we give an answer and that's it. We have a tendency to want to skip to the end of any story just so that we can get to the bottom line and move on to the next thing. So, like my friend, I really didn't take much pleasure from sitting around having idle conversation with my woman because very little of what she was saying had enough substance to be of interest to me. But over time I've learned that there is a compromise to be made here, because lending an ear to our counterpart for the smallest amount of time can save a lot of grief and headaches. Let me give you an example.

During the course of my third marriage, I was in a situation where I was working between forty-eight and sixty hours a week while going to school full-time. My typical schedule went about like this: I would wake up at 6:00 in the evening to be at work by 7:00. I worked twelve-hour shifts from 7:00 at night until 7:00 in the morning, at which point I would leave work going straight to class which began at 8:00 am. Classes lasted until 11:45 am, which meant that I wouldn't get home until about 12:30 in the afternoon. I would walk in the house, say "hello", eat something, and go to bed so that I could get **maybe** five hours of sleep before I had to get up and do it all over again.

What that normally got me was some type of attitude from my wife when I woke up, which ultimately resulted in an argument as I was running out the door trying to beat rush-hour traffic so as not to be late for work. Let me share with you a typical conversation of one of these arguments in order to explain the differences in both of our reasonings.

I would say, "Baby, you know I'm not doing all of this just for me; I'm working to take care of our family and going to school so that I can provide an even better life for all of us in the future!"

Her response to this was, "I understand all of that, but what you are missing is that all I seem to get of you is the leftovers. I don't even get to *talk* to you!"

Damned if I do...damned if I don't!

So what I began to do was to take about fifteen or twenty minutes as soon as I got home (after changing my clothes, but before eating, because you know food will put you right to sleep) to talk to my wife about whatever she wanted. And you know what? As it turned out, she didn't want **me** to talk at all. She just wanted me to listen to what was going on with her, and appear as though I was paying attention.

Although I must admit that most of the time I wasn't.

Evidently, this woman had a subconscious need, once the evening had begun, to verbalize all of the chronological events of that particular day and any consequent realizations that may have occurred to her during that time. Therefore, me having to engage in actual conversation was a moot point, and thus, something that I could easily handle. When I was really tired, I could just sit there and look directly into her eyes and say "Uh-huh...", "Oh, really?", and "Oh okay, Baby." for about fifteen minutes or so and she was just as content as could be. Subsequently, the attitudes and arguments when I woke up were replaced with warm smiles and kisses before I left.

Who knew?!

Now fellas, don't mistake what I'm saying to mean that you should fake listening to your lady while intentionally ignoring everything that she is saying. I <u>had</u> to do that occasionally just to get a somewhat sufficient amount of sleep. And, doing so **will** come back to haunt you because at some point she will ask you about something that she has said to you while you were "faking it", and you won't have the slightest clue as to what she is talking about.

"But Honey", she'll say, " I just told you this morning that I thought we should do such and such, and you said okay…how can you not remember?"

And you'll look at her like a deer in headlights! BUSTED!! What I am saying is that women **need** to be able to talk to us…they require it. And although it's not part of the average man's basic make-up to be an intense listener, if we want to keep a relationship strong…we should lend one another our ear on a regular basis. Trust me. I know that is a tall order to fill for a lot of us because for the most part, men and women don't enjoy talking about the same things. You see, I've come to realize that men and women think differently, we hear things differently; so therefore when we decide to talk to each other, we naturally do that differently as well. Most of the time, the subjects that interests each of the genders are worlds apart. Men like to talk about things that are exact, concrete, and factual like hunting, sports, and tools. These are the conversations to which there are no questions: like when a team wins a football game by ten points; that is a definitive victory over an opponent by a specific margin. Or, when two twelve-inch pieces of wood have to be nailed together at a ninety degree angle; that is raw material that we can hold in our hand that has to be configured to a precise measurement. These are the types of issues that are attractive to the literal brains of the male species. Now most women, on the other hand, like to talk about things that are creative, open-ended, and emotional. Shopping, soap operas, and matters of the heart are all figurative topics of conversations that ladies relish in, and most guys try to avoid like the Bubonic plague. But nonetheless, these conversations are important to our relationships. Although the subject matter with which our spouse is trying to engage us may not be able to stir the slightest inkling of interest on our part, it is still his/her way of sharing themselves with us through the act of speech. I've finally come to an understanding that it's not the topic of the conversation that should be important to me; it is the bearer of it.

Now, there's one other major point about communication that I want to mention because it took me a long time to figure this out for myself. And that is that men and women speak in <u>two</u> different languages (kinda like French and Spanish). Although both of our words sound the same, the meanings can sometimes be totally opposite. That's because we guys use logic as the basis of our conversation because we are programmed to think in literal terms; and women, on the other hand, reason in a more figurative manner and therefore use emotions as the source of their lingo. Try this scenario for an example. When a lady asks her man how she looks in a particular outfit, he will (like most men) assume that she wants his honest input. Simple logic leads him to believe that if he tells her that the outfit is "a little snug" around the mid-section, she can change into something else before going out in public; and he's just saved the day. Right?
Wrong!!

No, the guy doesn't even have a chance at this one because he doesn't understand the question…it was asked in another language. The man hears "Honey, how do I look in this outfit?" But translated into "woman-ese", that means "Honey, I'm not getting too fat, am I?" You see what I mean? She knew the outfit was too tight when she was looking at herself in the mirror. But, in a state of feminine physical preservation, she came to her man seeking emotional reassurance about her outward attractiveness. And he just failed her…miserably. He couldn't help it though, because as I've said a couple of times now, a man's discourse is logical and a women's is emotional. However, I made up this lighthearted scenario to demonstrate a very important point.

I promise you ladies, I have never told a woman that she was too fat…that story was completely fictional!

There have been numerous occasions where I have had a normal conversation with my significant other turn into an all out argument, and the reason was that we were communicating on two totally different levels. Actually, I would dare say that most arguments that we have with our counterparts are due to this difference in the male and female diction. The problem seems to be that we men feel that woman should think like us; and of course, women feel men should think like them. So when we are talking to one another, there is the expectation that the other person should not only understand what we are saying, but agree with it as well. Somehow, when this does not happen, each of the participating members are genuinely surprised, at which point they take the course of action to attempt to convince the other constituent to see things "their way".

Does this sound familiar to anybody?

Yeah, this is the wonderful world of communication that our heavenly creator envisioned for Adam and Eve. So I ask you – would you like to know what the solution is for this ageless obstacle between the sexes? Good…please be sure to enlighten me if you should happen to find out because this is one of those divine solutions that still escapes me to this day. But, what I have found is that sometimes just knowing that a difference exists can help bridge the gap in our conversation by making us a little bit more understanding. I mean, if you were forced to have a relationship with a person that spoke a language other than English, what would you do? Would you not talk to them at all or figure out an alternative method of communicating with them. It's pretty much the same concept between the sexes.

Except there's no translation dictionary that we can refer to when there's something we don't understand.

I think we have to be willing to stand in there and give an effort to get past all of the smokescreens and figure out a way to get through to one another on the important stuff. Yeah, I know; it seems like it shouldn't have to be so complicated, but it usually is. And if you should happen to be fortunate enough to be with a person with whom you like talking to and can communicate with easily, consider yourself blessed; because for most of us, that's not the case. There is a daily journey between most couples to find common ground on which they can comprehend and empathize with one another in the art of verbal expression. But don't give up, my newfound friends, because I have come to an absolute certainty that communication is the lifeline of any relationship. Those types of conversations that I mentioned when we began this chapter are essential to the lines of communication between us and our beloved. The time that we spend with our significant other will be much more fulfilling if we put in the necessary work to keep those vital lines of communication open.

I'm just the friendly switchboard operator trying to connect two parties who want to talk!

IV: Togetherness

It seems to me that this subject is the one individual part of any typical relationship that is the easiest to get lost. As human beings, we have a natural instinct to satisfy our individual needs and desires before attending to those of others. But that is one of those things that is supposed to change whenever we enter into any serious relationship, especially marriage, because we are committing ourselves to become part of a single unit. We are making a conscious agreement to be accountable to another person in any and every action we take from this point forward. Now please don't misunderstand me; I'm not saying that there is not a place for independence in a relationship between a man and woman, because there is. I believe that the man should have his life and the woman should have hers, and together they share their lives with each other. I mean, each and every one of us has had dreams and desires that motivated us to greater aspirations long before we became a participating part of "a couple". And those dreams and desires are the very things that make us who we are, and normally the same things that attract another person to us in the first place. So I have an adamant belief that no one should ever have to give up who they <u>are</u> because of who they are <u>with</u>.
Remember? I came to this conclusion back in "Self-Understanding" when this was an on-going problem for me.

The trick, in my opinion, is to be able to maintain our own identity while still being able to identify with our spouse; and in a perfect world, those individual characteristics will compliment one another. In order to accomplish this, I've learned that we more or less have to be willing to treat our relationship with our significant other almost like a business partnership. I know that probably sounds kind of strange, but I've also been in quite a few business partnerships and I can assure you that there are numerous parallels between the joint ventures in business and the partnerships of love. When I say that, I mean that the two people must both have the same vision, it is essential that they be able to communicate with one another (which we talked about earlier), and they most certainly must be able to accomplish things by working together. Just like in the corporate office, at home there should be "board meetings" (family conversations), financial reviews, and most important, the ability to work as a team. And to me, that's the key! I am truly convinced that most successful relationships have this one thing in common – the two people that are participating in the relationship must almost always be working on something together. And for each couple the choice will be different, obviously, because every union has a core set of interests that are unique to them. It can be sharing projects that are as simple as exercising or dieting together to get in shape, to ones as complex as finding a new home to purchase. Once one goal has been achieved, then the subsequent step for the couple should be to determine what the next project will be, and then start working on the preliminary plans to accomplish it. I have found that to have some type of coherent effort between partners at any given time is almost a necessity. Now sometimes our projects will not necessarily involve both people at the same time. For instance, one person might be working to accomplish a mission that is specific to them, while the other simply offers support when and where it is needed. But even that support keeps us close in our thoughts and efforts, and helps to prevent the possibility of unwanted distance – which plagues so many couples – from creeping in unexpectedly. Case and point. My third wife and I decided that we wanted to improve the appearance of the house that we were living in at the time by collectively undertaking a couple of "do-it-yourself" projects. Now I need you to understand that I was not necessarily what you would call an "interior decorator", and I definitely didn't have the desire to become one! But she was a good sport about that; and besides, she wanted the pleasure of remodeling the inside of the house to herself anyway. And she took it on with a passion like you wouldn't believe! Now while this was really <u>her</u> project, I did do things like providing money for any of the new furniture that she wanted; arranging to have it picked up and then moving it into the house; and finally, putting anything together that did not come already pre-assembled.

You know the "guy" stuff!

And although I tried my best on each and every occasion to get out of it, sometimes I would even have to go with her to the department store to give my opinion on drapes and decorations and bathroom sets and all of those little things that ironically would have to be decided on whenever the weekend's football games were on.

*And of course, all guys no how much fun **that** can be!*

But she labored with an undaunted intensity; and it was always funny to me whenever she had placed a new piece of furniture or finished a certain room, and I would have to step outside of that particular room and then step in again in order to get the "wow" effect! And I must admit, that at the end of all of this intense (and at times, crazy) reconstruction, she had done a fabulous job with the project and I actually enjoyed coming home to feel the new ambiance that she had created in our house. There were pretty drapes that matched the carpet, and sofa tables with dainty antique telephones, and curios and oil paintings – the list goes on – and these were all pleasantries that a simple guy like me would have never taken the initiative to obtain. But, she was a woman to whom it was important to have a house that drew people's attention while still making them feel comfortable; and I was happy to help her achieve that. However, once she felt like she had come as close to finishing the remodeling of our home as space (and our budget) would allow, it was now time for me to begin my project of landscaping our yard. Don't be fooled though; because just as I'm no interior decorator, neither have I ever had much of a "green thumb". My father and my grandmother (my mom's mom) were both very good with planting and raising things, but somehow none of those talents happened to filter down to yours truly. But the project was fun for me because I was determined to match (if not outdo) her with the "guy's" portion of the improvements that were being made to our home. Along the way, I also learned a lot of stuff like how to aerate a yard, plant grass and shrubbery, put down mulch…that sort of thing.

And I must confess here that a nice father-in-law is a good thing to have, because this particular one helped me figure out most of this stuff; so while I put in most of the work, I cannot in good conscience take all of the credit.

And although I didn't actually develop a "green thumb" during this project, I believe I did quite well.

And my thumb is now a little yellowish.

I got that human satisfaction that we all enjoy when we achieve something that we've never attempted before. And the togetherness was still accomplished because my wife had lent her support throughout this process by going with me to help pick out plants and shrubbery; by making sure that the sprinkler system was turned on for me at night when I wasn't there to do it; and sometimes, even standing outside and watching me while I was planting, digging, and raking…and getting all tired and sweaty.

Big help there! No, really she would cheer me on, make sure that I didn't get too hot, and bring me stuff to drink when I needed it.

Anyway, once that was all said and done, I believe we were drawn closer together by the fact that our teamwork had produced the absolute best looking house, both inside and out, in our neighborhood. And the resulting closeness was the most important achievement of all because that was one of those singular periods in that marriage that stand out to me as a time when we were the most connected to one another. We were both involved and focused on the same thing, and therefore we were both involved and focused on each other. It was the togetherness that I spoke of earlier, which made us individually feel that we were part of a whole.

Now please keep in mind, the projects between you and your mate may be much simpler (and less exhaustive) than mine was; but anything that keeps two people working together towards a common objective should produce similar results. It can be as simple as participating in a mutual hobby such as bowling together or even having a joint preparation of each day's evening meal. As I said in the opening statement of this chapter, the act of being together is something that is often easily lost in the hustle and bustle of everyday life because we simply take it for granted. We just assume that because we see one another every day in passing – while getting dressed in the morning for work or watching a television show over dinner – that it is enough to constitute the idea of always being together. But I submit that there has to be more work involved than that; I believe that there has to be a conscious effort placed on not only the amount of time we spend with our counterpart, but what that time with them is spent doing. It is important – no, actually it is essential to the healthiness of any relationship because it is during these times of togetherness that we are able to share with one another the details of the life that we are maintaining whenever we are apart.

Remember, I did say earlier that we are still entitled to our independence? This is how I think all of that ties in together.

It is during these times that we are able to make the most significant strides towards bringing the two individual worlds that we each existed in, prior to the current romantic collaboration, together to become the one universe which we share for the mutual benefit of happiness. I have found that taking the time to sit down with my lady and express to her all of my individual goals, and then allowing her the opportunity to share the same with me, can work wonders in a relationship. We tend to find out that there are a lot of things that the two of us can do together; and if not, then our counterpart might simply be able to provide the support base that we may need to achieve our individual goals, just because they know up front what it is we are attempting to accomplish. And on the flip side, we have to be committed to put forth the same effort into being just as attentive and supportive of their goals and desires as well. This way, even if there are not always "joint ventures" to work on, both individuals can continue to bounce back and forth between each of their separate endeavors. And that is what

I think keeps us interacting on a common ground; and as I said earlier, when two people are involved and focused on the same thing, then they usually are involved and focused on each other as well.

I have come to believe that in any relationship, the two people should have similar goals and objectives. Whenever that is the case, it normally allows for us to have enough of the same interest together to keep us operating within a realm of commonality. I also believe that whenever this state of unity is not a natural occurrence or ceases to exist, it is essential that we make the effort to work as a team in order to create it. I truly believe that doing things together produces <u>togetherness</u>. And you know what? That's really what it's all about! Isn't the primary reason we seek companionship is to have a "lifelong partner"…or that "other half"…or the person that will always "have our back"? Isn't the whole point of all of this madness we call love to find that person that we can journey through this life with and at the end, look back on all we've been able to accomplish – together? Call me crazy, but it's the only way I want it! And I'd be willing to bet, that no one would be listening to anything "the professional husband" has to say if almost everyone out there didn't want the same…to be <u>together</u>, forever!

V: Romance

Oooooh yeah...romance! This element of any union is the one that is the most fun, especially for me because I am a hopeless romantic. But I've concluded that this may be largely due to the fact that I watched too much television while I was growing up; and in my house, the television was predominately controlled by women. "*All My Children*", "*One Life To Live*" during the day and "*Dynasty*" and "*Dallas*" at night; you name it – if there was hugging, kissing, emotions, and drama involved, then it was on the television somewhere in the Thomas family household.

And to all the guys who are reading this – I don't watch soap operas anymore...in case you might have been wondering. Although I do happen to still think that J.R. Ewing was a pretty cool dude.

Nonetheless, as a man, this is the part in a relationship that we can actually enjoy as much as the women. And, in case you didn't know, romance is our trump card when we get in trouble with our lady (which I've had a lot of practice doing).

Come on...tell me that a dozen roses or a candlelit dinner has never gotten any of you other guys out of the doghouse before? Yeah, now you see my point.

But romance could, and should, be about more than having a convenient "get-out-of-jail-free" card. Romance is the essence of why men and women get together in the first place...it's the embodiment of the attraction, the passion, and the intimacy that draws the opposite sexes to one another. The secret is to make sure that romance remains a healthy part of a relationship so that the two parties have the emotional desire to actually stay together. Now like I mentioned a minute ago, I have always been, and am still now, a hopeless romantic, so I tend to think that I am pretty good at expressing my romantic side to women. I can honestly say that this romantic nature of mine is probably the one strength that I have which has allowed me to experience my numerous relationships with women. Lord knows that without it, half of them probably wouldn't have given me the time of day, much less hang around long enough to end up married or engaged to me. Check out one of my stories…

Once upon a marriage, my wife and I were about to have our first wedding anniversary; and I had decided that I would go all out for this one (which is probably the reason why I remember it in particular, considering how many different ones I've had). I began by calling the hotel where our wedding reception had been held and reserving the exact same suite that she and I had stayed in the night we got married. Next, I ordered a stretch limousine to chauffer us around for our night out; and not one of those cheap ones – I'm talking about a ten-passenger white stretch limousine complete with champagne in the back. Finally, I made reservations at the most elaborate and romantic restaurant that I could think of in the city. This place was exquisite with a capital "E" – it had a dim lobby with the sitting area around a brick fireplace. And once inside the dining area, there was an ambience to die for!

Oh yeah, the meal cost me more than a day's pay; but it was worth every penny!

So, everything was set. Early that brisk morning of our anniversary, I left the house and informed her that I would be back to pick her up at 6:30 p.m. sharp and that she should be dressed and standing outside when I got there. Of course, she inquired as to how she needed to be dressed for the evening, and when I told her to select the most elegant of the dresses or evening gowns she possessed, you could see on her face the anticipation that was obviously welling up inside. From home, I went out to pick up everything I would need for the night and then went to set up our hotel room. I labored the entire day trying to get everything just right; and finally, once I was satisfied that perfection had been accomplished, I got all dressed up in the finest evening suit that I owned.

Reminded me of the way my dad used to do. And I must say that I think I looked rather dashing…if I do say so myself!

Well, at precisely 6:00 p.m., the limo arrived for me at the hotel and with a dash, we were off to pick up the lady of the evening. And there she was – outside in front of our house talking to the neighbors when I pulled up in this long, pearl-white limousine. And as it came to stop, I got out (as if from a horse-driven carriage) and handed her a single rose…her knight in shining armor. The dreamy smile that was on her face as we drove away was more than enough proof for me that I had done well! When we got to the restaurant for dinner, our driver asked us to stay in the car while he announced our arrival to the restaurant and he would come get us when it was time to be seated!

You know I ended up tipping that guy really well, because he absolutely made me look like a superstar!

As we sat in the car, all of the people who were walking by tried to get a glimpse of who these "important people" were inside of this limo parked in front of the restaurant. They had to be thinking, "Must be somebody famous…or somebody really rich."

Nope – it's just little ol' me in all of my romantic glory!

And my wife was soaking up every bit of this attention that I was laying on her so thickly. Once inside, we were fortunate enough to be seated on one the plush sofas in the lobby that was right next to that beautiful fireplace, where we enjoyed a fabulous glass of wine together. Shortly thereafter, we were ushered to our table and we savored an exquisite meal in this fabulous atmosphere; and then it was back to the limo for a ride around the city at night. The limousine ride was just as magical as we sipped champagne and toured the city as though we had never lived there before.

We did, however, have to stop off at one of her friend's house so that she could show off her husband and the magnificent evening that he was giving her.

We also stopped in the heart of downtown and enjoyed a nice quiet walk along the river…just the two of us. Finally, our chariot delivered us back to the hotel and she was absolutely flabbergasted when she realized where we were staying and what suite we would be in. I thanked the driver immensely and proceeded to lead her upstairs to the suite that would be our final destination for the evening. Once she was settled in, I served her strawberries that I had injected with pink champagne and dipped in chocolate earlier that day, before allowing them to chill. Now because it was in fact winter, she inquired as to where I had gotten strawberries; and was overly impressed to find out that I had had them flown in from California.

Which between you and I only means that I had gone to a local produce dealer and the guy charged me twelve bucks to have a pint of strawberries added to his next shipment coming in from the West Coast! But hey, it sounded better my way.

As we sat on the couch curled up together eating chocolate covered strawberries and sipping champagne, I inconspicuously pressed "PLAY" on the VCR (which I had also set up earlier in the day), which immediately began showing the tape of our wedding and reception that I had brought from home; and we blissfully reminisced about the day exactly one year ago that had led us to this actual celebration. Afterwards, I drew for her a hot bath with honey-and-milk scented bubbles in the oversized tub and lit all twenty of the candles that I had strategically positioned around it.

Hey; I told you I worked all day on this!
On the way from the living room to her bath, she couldn't help but notice that I had covered the king-sized bed with an ornate amount of fresh rose pedals; and I can't say for sure, but I think her legs buckled a little bit when I mentioned that I had hand picked the pedals from the roses myself! But at this point, I'm going to end this particular story because it's not my desire to be writing one of those hot and steamy romance novels…and plus some things should just be left to the imagination. Nevertheless, I share this experience with you to not only prove beyond a shadow of a doubt that I know a little bit about romance, but to also set the tone for my thoughts on its importance in a relationship.

One of the important things I've learned throughout all of my amorous quests is that romance is even more than just thoughtful and loving gestures like the elaborate one that I just replayed for you. I've found that when we take the time to ensure its place in any worthwhile relationship, it can be the catalyst for a connection between souls and the language for an unspoken love. By that I mean that romance is the component that can allow a man and woman to say "I love you" to one another from across a crowded room without ever opening their mouth – they can accomplish it through simple eye contact! Romance is the thing that turns your intimacy from mere sex into the ultimate sharing of one another at the deepest levels of your souls. Romance is...well, it is the means of actually expressing true love because sometimes just saying it isn't enough. I mean, there have been plenty of instances when I have been involved with a lady and she has professed her undying love for me. But for whatever reason, I could not feel the love from her that she was verbally expressing.

And isn't that what we all yearn for...to "feel" loved?
I truly believe that because love is an emotion, it should be demonstrated from one person to another through emotional acts; not just through mere words. And in every relationship, it has to be something that is felt and not just heard. And I have come to realize, that romance is the human method of putting that love into wordless expressions. It is the act of showing a person that is special to us how we feel about them, so that saying it to them is merely a gesture of confirmation. And, I have learned from this realization to be cautious never to let the romance fade away...never to let the flame die out.

Now, because romance is enjoyable to both parties in a relationship, it should never really be hard to accomplish; and it doesn't always have to be overly elaborate or expensive. Gentlemen, sometimes picking up a single rose on the way home from work can go a long way.
You'll spend three dollars, max.
Or giving her a passionate kiss or a long hug can make her day (and your night, if you know what I mean).
For you ladies, most of us guys are enamored by a nice massage when we come home from work. And one of my personal favorites is the exhibition of erotic lingerie just before it's time for bed.

Hey, I'm a guy and we are not that hard to please!

It's really not that important what we choose to do, just as long as we choose to do something! I find it difficult to understand when people tell me that "the romance is gone" from their relationship. Romance is not something that can come and go in a relationship, it's something you bring to it! Whenever people say that to me, I have to believe that they just weren't trying hard enough. Romance has always been the fuel for relationships. And just as with any other machine we deal with, when our relationship's "tank" is starting to get close to empty, we have to refill it; otherwise we won't go very far. And for as much traveling as I have done on the highways of love, I've learned to keep my romance "tank" as close to full as possible. As is probably not hard for you to believe, I've actually come to somewhat cherish my romantic side; because without it, I don't know where I'd be today. But I sure wouldn't be here as a professional husband writing this book!

VI: Respect

It's kind of hard for me to pick one particular place to begin when it comes to talking about respect. I mean, I've had so much trouble trying to get this right, Aretha Franklin thought she'd help me out by writing a song for me back in the 60's.
R-E-S-P-E-C-T! Maybe you've heard it?
Anyway, I must say that I think respect is one of, if not the most, complex issues involved in having a relationship because it ties into so many of the other components that we deal with. I've learned that it not only has to do with the basic idea of two people having to respect one another as individuals (and more specifically as a man or woman), but it also filters down to respecting each other's feelings as well. From there, it seems that respecting one another's space comes into play; and then that leads into being able respect the other person's belongings – and the list goes on and on and on. Now, I can't possibly take the time to go into the details of each and every one of these aspects regarding this topic, but I do want to touch on a few critical realizations that have come to me over the years because I feel that respect serves as an undertone to the foundation of any relationship. So, I'll try to stick to the basics.
Deal?

I've often heard people say that respect is not something that is given; it is something that is earned. And while I do believe that this phrase has a certain degree of logic to it, I have a tendency not to agree with it entirely because I do not believe that it is an absolute truth. I believe that respect is something that <u>should</u> be given…that if I show you respect, then you'll show respect to me in return. I have the optimistic notion that it is a natural courtesy that intelligent creatures extend to one another with the assumption that the sentiment will be reciprocated. Now we all know that this is not always the case and that people will disrespect us sometimes for no real reason at all. And that is usually where problems begin; especially with us men, who have historically been notorious for overreacting when it comes to the issue of respect (or the lack thereof).

Tell the truth – how many fights have you ever seen started based on the words "He was trying to disrespect me!"?

But even still, I've found that taking the chance to give others respect is the most probable way to get it from them in return. And it has been my experience that there is no other situation where this is more true than in a relationship between a man and woman. Respect is one of those things I feel that we should give our mate as freely as we give them our love. I have not always felt this way; but I do believe that since the period in which I began to appreciate this emotion, I have been able to avoid some of the many pitfalls that have plagued my coexistence with women. And on that note, you know I have a story to tell.

During my third marriage, my wife and I seemed to develop a nasty little tendency to argue quite frequently. And as you might be able to imagine, the more routine the arguments became, the more severe they became. We ultimately found ourselves in the habit of being disrespectful in our arguments by calling each other out of our names and saying other hurtful things to one another. Needless to say, this was one of the downfalls to that marriage; but before the two of us decided to call it quits, we did attempt to try to resolve the problem through counseling. And while counseling did seem to help a little, I think that we were too far gone by the time we got there. Yet, there were a few positive things that I was able to take away from those weekly sessions; and one of them was that arguments are a natural, and even healthy, part of any relationship. However, there are rules to successfully having them in a correct way in order to maintain the respect between the arguing parties.

Imagine that! Rules for arguing?
The counselor said that one of the first rules of successfully having an argument is that you should never let it get to a point where hurtful and disrespectful things are said back and forth to each other. The use of vulgar language and the calling of names are absolute no-no's! Our counselor told us that whenever this becomes the case, then the individuals should take a break from the argument and then resume it again later when both parties can speak their minds in at least a respectful manner. He went on to explain that the reason this happens is because our bodies are chemically designed to produce adrenaline whenever it feels the threat of attack; however, our glands are incapable of telling the difference between an all out physical attack and merely a verbal one. So, when there is no physical threat to channel that adrenaline to (hopefully), it manifests itself in the form of an aggressive verbal mechanism – hence, the name calling and vulgar language become a form of retaliation.

That's pretty deep, huh?
And there were quite a few other things that the counselor went on to explain about the subject, but the main point that I took away is that two people should try very hard to never be in a situation where they are disrespecting one another by saying or doing hurtful things. This is important because every time we allow this to happen, we chip away at the

core of all the good things in our relationship. Each time we say something that is hurtful to our spouse, although they may forgive us, it stays with them. And it ultimately piles on to all of the other nasty things that have been said; to the point where it's festering…it's chipping away at their feelings us. And if we do that enough times, ultimately there'll be nothing left to "chip away" at. So I've learned to be cautious in regards to talking to my significant other in a respectful manner, even when we are angry. I realize that while my counselor may have given a good explanation as to why disrespectful things fly out of my mouth, he couldn't tell me how to take them back or remove the damage that they cause.

Okay, I want to talk about one other aspect of this particular subject and it deals with respecting one another's feelings. This has proven to be a very hard concept for me to grasp because, I must admit, for most of my life I have been fairly selfish and didn't really place a priority on other people's feelings. As it turns out, that is not a desirable trait when it comes to participating in an intimate partnership with another person. But this book is about all of the things that I've learned from my mistakes, and this subject is to be no different. Although it took me quite some time to actually understand this concept, I think that I have finally gotten better at it. And of course there's a story to tell; but this one now seems so trivial, I'm almost ashamed to share it with you. But you know I'm going to anyway! So to begin, we have to again refer to Wife #3…

Actually I'm pretty sure that I had this problem with Wives #1 & #2 as well, but #3 was the one who helped correct the problem.

As I mentioned in the previous story, it seems like this woman and I were always arguing.

Do you think that was a sign of some sort?
When I think back, I can't remember whose fault it was most of the time; but it didn't really matter because I had this annoying habit of anytime she would get mad or upset at me about something, I would automatically get mad too. I don't know why I did it, but I'm certain that I can't be the only person who's ever been guilty of this.
I'm hoping it's another one of those defense mechanisms or something...kinda like the adrenaline theory that my counselor gave me! If that's not it, the only other thing I can come up with is that I was just being childish. Naaaah, not me!
But anyway, it was always a certainty that if she was mad, then so was I. And each and every time this happened, sure enough we would end up in a huge argument...normally for something that started out small. And finally one day, in the middle of her anger (and mine) this groundbreaking conversation hit me dead in the face.

She asked me, "Why can't I ever just be mad all by myself?"

Now this is a question you don't hear everyday, so to buy some time, I replied, "What's that supposed to mean?"

She answered, "Do you realize that if I'm mad at you about something, you have to be mad too? Why can't you respect my feelings enough to let me be mad all by myself? If you would just let me talk about whatever it is that's bothering me, then that would probably be the end of it. But instead, you get mad at me– just because I'm mad – and we end up having some big stupid argument that's not even necessary!"
Whoa! Really?

So at this point, I'm having another one of my "deer-in-the-headlights" moments. I mean, when you look at it that way, me being mad made no sense at all. I could have

given her ten minutes of madness all by herself, and then I could have been on my way?
Why can't everything be that easy for guys?
Now I like to think of myself as a pretty smart guy, so for the life of me, I can't understand why I couldn't have figured that one out on my own. But at this point, it doesn't even matter – lesson learned! I now realize that there is something to be said about respecting a person enough to allow them their feelings and then granting them the ability to express them without repercussions. And seriously, I hope that this is a brief, but valuable lesson of respecting one another's feelings that can be learned by everyone.

I know that there are many more facets to the subject of respect, but I chose these two because they are the areas where I appear to have made the most progress. You would think the concept of showing respect in the things that you do and say to someone, as well as being able to respect their feelings, are lessons that my mother would have taught me.
Which she did, I just don't think I was paying attention!
Sorry, Mama!
But as adults, we tend to overlook these elementary sentiments between one another; and this is especially true in our romantic interactions. If you will remember, earlier I referred to respect as an undertone in the foundation of our relationships. I'd like to expand on that by explaining that respect is very rarely the main topic when we are dealing with the intimate details of our amorous correlations; but it's always there – underneath the surface of everything else that we hold dear. It is a part of how we communicate with one another; it is a part of how we treat one another; and it is, without a doubt, a part of how we love one another. We should show respect for our mates; we should show respect for our relationships; and we should most importantly show

respect for ourselves. All of these are the lessons that I have learned through much heartache and chagrin. Unfortunately, learning these lessons have not come without a price; they have come at the expense of having hurt some of the people for whom I have cared deeply. I trust that in sharing these experiences, someone, somewhere, might be spared the heartache of being disrespected by a person they love. If that is the case, then perhaps I have made some atonement for the sins of my past.

VII: Trust

I know that this particular subject will probably cause quite a few mixed emotions as you read this chapter because it is a topic that usually has varying degrees of opinions, according to the individual. Let me begin by saying that I believe that trust is a hard enough attribute to accomplish in the simplest of relationships (for example; friends, family, coworkers, etc.), much less in the more complex and intimate one between a man and woman. And the reason for this is that trust involves the voluntary act of placing oneself in a state of vulnerability; and as human beings, we naturally try to avoid allowing ourselves to become prone to that particular condition. It is a natural instinct for people to engage the mechanism of self-preservation in order to protect ourselves from any outside force that can in any way cause harm to our well-being. In spite of this mortal characteristic, I think that the more intimate a relationship becomes between two people, the more trust they will allow themselves to extend; thus the more vulnerable they will allow themselves to become. Now I, being a professional husband and all, have found myself exceptionally vulnerable to the act of having to trust people on many occasions, and have therefore had to come to my own rationalizations about how to best deal with this particular emotion. My personal definition of trust is this: the belief someone holds that a person, thing, or circumstance will meet the expectations that they have

placed upon it and not cause disappointment, regret, or emotional pain.
I didn't take the time to look up Webster's definition for this, but you are more than welcome to if you don't particularly like mine.
In other words, whenever I sit down in a chair, I am placing my trust in that particular piece of furniture. I am believing that it will meet the expectations of the manufacturer to hold me up and not let me come crashing down to the floor, thereby regretting that I ever attempted to sit in it in the first place. As simplistic as that may sound, I feel that it is the same way with relationships. Think about it; we are expecting the person in which we are placing this trust to meet our expectations of loving us, standing by us, making us happy, and being true and faithful to us. We are trusting them not to leave us, abuse us, or cheat on us, and thereby hurting us to the point where we wished we had never taken a chance on them at all. Now I'd like to make an interjection here to say that I believe love plays a big part of trust and the more you love someone, the more you expect these things to hold true – **and** the more vulnerable you become.

Now, I know that my version of having to trust someone in a relationship probably sounds morbid and scary, but it really is not. In my various escapades in heterosexual intimacy, I have determined that trust is a very simple and wonderful part of romantic relations between the goose and the gander. When I say that, I mean that in a way, trust is the easiest way to gauge the soundness of a relationship. For instance, I believe that we can tell when we are starting to fall in love with someone because it seems as though that person can do no wrong in our eyes. "Working late" means working late and "out with some friends" means out with some friends! And that's the way it **should** be because every relationship between two people who love each other is supposed to have a trust with no limits. Unfortunately, there is a thing called "life" that does from time to time test this trust, and ultimately will place limits on it and sometimes even break it. Going back to what I mentioned earlier, I would now like to point out how trust becomes a good measure of the status of a relationship. I think that once the trust has limitations, then so does the relationship; once the trust is broken, then, I believe, so is the relationship. And most of the time, we as mortals don't intentionally harm the trust; it occurs from things as inconsequential as making a devastating comment during an argument that deeply hurts our significant other or developing agendas that are so isolated between the two of us that neither person supports the other. While on the surface these things seem like "the cost of doing business" when it comes to love, the reality is that if we can't trust our better half to in some way participate in the achievement of our goals or trust them to respect us as a person in the way they talk to us, then we will naturally become reluctant to trust them with any of the deeper matters of our soul. I have experienced both of these scenarios firsthand (and from both sides of the fence), and I can honestly attest to the damage that is ultimately left behind in a relationship. And then there's the granddaddy of all the trust-breakers – infidelity.

I use that word because it obviously sounds better than cheating or adultery; which should give you an idea that I've committed this act at some point and time because of my sensitivity to the way it is characterized.

I must tell you now that I personally think that once infidelity is introduced into a relationship, it's a deal-breaker. Now I know that there have been many cases where someone has gotten caught with their pants down (literally), and the relationship survived. But these are **my** personal thoughts and I can say from **my** personal experience that I believe these instances to be in the minority in today's society. I believe that while the trust between two people can be rebuilt after the act of unfaithfulness, it can never be the same as it was before the act occurred. And I believe that this goes back to the vulnerability factor because once a person's trust has been broken, they will never allow themselves to be as vulnerable as they were before; therefore they will never trust the other person in quite the same way because that person has shown the capacity to cause hurt. I mean let's face it, when it comes to infidelity there is no such thing as a mistake or an accident.

"Oooops! I'm sorry. I was just walking along minding my own business, and wouldn't you know it - I accidentally tripped on something and fell into that other person's bed by mistake...on accident...mistakenly!"

No matter what the situation (even being in an intoxicated state), a person makes a conscious decision (never mind if it's a faulty one) to engage in the pleasures of the flesh with someone other than their exclusive counterpart. And while it may be considered a <u>bad</u> decision, it was a **decision** nonetheless...not a mistake or accident. As I said before, there are those people who can rebuild trust between them once this occurs, but I think that they are few and far between; and even then, that trust is not the same unadulterated type of conviction that existed before. Let me give you an example. Remember Fiancé #2 who lived in New Jersey? Well, while were engaged, we often went a couple of weeks without seeing each other due to the distance. And there was this one particular instance where we had not shared one another's company in over a month. Now it was during this exact period of time that a certain co-worker of the female persuasion had begun to make intimate advances towards me. And I, being a young, virile man at that time, decided to playfully entertain those advances of this particular co-worker of the female persuasion and – well, you can use your imagination for the rest.

And honestly folks, I really only had the intentions of doing a little flirting and things just kinda got out of hand. But, you know that I'm true to my word; so I cannot say it was a mistake; I made a bad decision.

And as luck would have it, two weeks later I was at my fiancé's house in New Jersey and happened to be checking the messages from my home phone; and just as I was listening to a message from "my co-worker of the female persuasion" about how she was missing me and wished that I were there with her, my fiancé inadvertently picked up the telephone in another room to make a call. I tried to get out of it, but this was the point where I learned that when you're caught, you're caught; and sometimes it's better to just tell the truth than to add insult to injury with a bad lie!

Really, I did learn my lesson from this!!

Needless to say that we went through the whole "How could you hurt me like this?", and the, "I'm sorry, I'll never do it again!" thing; and believe it or not, she actually stayed with me.

With the condition that I promise never to see the other woman again, throw away my mattress, and quit my job! Now I grant you...not seeing the other woman was a reasonable request. But I ask you, was I honestly supposed to endure sleeping on the floor and having to forgo paying my bills?

Well, as time went by, I tried to work my way back into my fiancé's good graces; but let me tell you, it was a losing battle. First of all, we lived three hundred miles away from each other and I was required to call her before I could go around the corner to the convenience store for a loaf of bread! And I had to call to check in five minutes later when I got back!

Now, I didn't mind tucking my tail between my legs for a while, but being subjected to the treatment of a child was a real test of my resolve.

On top of that, any time I did not answer my phone when she would call, I had to undergo an interrogation equivalent to that of the Federal Bureau of Investigations. But I endured because I knew that I had been wrong and that I wanted to try to keep this woman in my life. Ultimately, though, it still didn't work; and while the subject of my cheating was not brought up as the reason for our no longer being able to live happily ever after, there is no question in my mind that it was the cancer that deteriorated the bond which we had once shared. The trust was gone and without it we couldn't survive. And thus, we fell victim to the Grim Reaper of unfaithfulness that had claimed so many relationships before us. So where am I going with all of this babbling about the "T" word?

Well, I think that if I had to characterize love as the heart of a relationship and communication as the bloodline, then trust would most certainly be the skeleton. Although you don't usually see it, it is what everything else is built around; it is what holds all of the other members together; it is what makes the whole able to move forward. I believe that trust should be cherished because it is something that is hard for another person to give. We should always be conscious that the person on the other side of the dinner table has made an emotional sacrifice to give us their trust and that their trust is a gift; and if we choose to abuse that gift through bad decisions and dire actions, then one day we will look across the table and that particular person won't be there.

Finally, I believe that trust is an absolute emotion…either you have it or you don't. I, personally, find no merit in "halfway" trusting someone because if what you feel is one-half trust, then the other half of your emotional sense is most certainly doubt. If your partner leaves the house and you have to try your hardest to believe they are going where they said they were, then that's not trust – that's hope…

You're hoping that they come back and don't break your heart today-
…and there's only a limited amount of happiness that can exist in that type of environment. My point is that just like love, trust is something that must be given in its entirety; otherwise it's not worth the effort. It's an emotion that we have to be willing to give to someone (no matter how vulnerable it makes us), as well as put forth the effort to deserve it from them in return. Yeah, I know that's a huge gamble to take with your heart, but take it from a guy who's rolled the dice of trust on numerous occasions – although your losses might at some point begin to seem unbearable, remember that the idea of finding that one big payoff always justifies rolling one more time!

VIII: Commitment

Uh-oh! Did I really dare bring up a conversation about commitment? Ooooh noooo! Everybody knows that guys are afraid of commitment – unless that guy happens to be a professional husband. And I would like to initiate this topic by stating that I personally think that saying all guys are afraid of commitment is far too broad of a statement; particularly because I believe that there is more than one kind of commitment when it comes to relationships.

I know by now it must be crossing your mind, "This guy doesn't make anything simple, does he?"

Well, I feel like there is a commitment to another person; and then there's a commitment to a relationship; and there's even a commitment to being committed. I know that sounds funny, but there is a point that I want to try to make if you will be so kind as to hear me out. I do not believe that men are any more afraid of commitment than women are; however, I do believe that sometimes both the male and female genders misunderstand the type of commitment that they are making and what is expected of them for making it.

See, I had a point after all.

So let's see if I can expand on that idea to help you understand my particular point of view on this subject.

In my travels, I've discovered that the first kind of commitment occurs at the very beginning stages of the relationship; during the phase when two people are getting to know each other for the first time. You know how the first date goes: there's a nice dinner, and maybe a movie or dancing afterward; and during this time, we're kinda feeling the person out and looking for a vibe that might lead to a second rendezvous. For me, this is a fairly simple type of commitment because all I am trying to do is determine whether or not this person has enough of the qualities I'm seeking to make me want to commit any significant amount of time pursuing a potential relationship with them. Now I, personally, don't believe that it should take more than two or three dates with someone to make this determination (and sometimes it may only take one date); but everyone is not a marital speedster like myself. For example, I have a buddy who would always date these women for about five or six months, and after all of that time, he would tell me that he wasn't even sure if he actually liked them. He would always give me these explanations such as he was waiting to see if it was going to turn into something or not. And normally, it did turn into something – a nightmare! But I could never understand how he could spend that kind of time with a person he wasn't even sure he liked enough to commit to some kind of relationship! Now I, on the other hand, spent a majority of the time on any of my <u>first</u> dates checking a woman out for marriage potential right from the start. It was always my intention to learn as much as possible about her religious values, her career ambitions, and her family plans for the future.

Hey, the application process is very important to a professional husband!

And if we weren't on the same wavelength on a majority of these issues, then at the end of the date I would recite to her the famous last words of Russell Simmons; "Thank you for coming out, God bless you, and good night!"
If you don't get that, then you have to go back and watch the old Def Comedy Jam series with Martin Lawrence.

But seriously, I've learned the importance of taking the time to decide early on if a new person in your life possesses the qualities, values, and attributes that we desire in a partner; because if they don't, then there's not much to try to build a relationship on (unless it's purely physical, and that conversation is the basis for an entirely separate chapter in what would be a sequel to this book), and the chances of failure are about ninety-nine percent. In that scenario, I would have to say that commitment is futile. But on the other hand, if we connect with a person during the first couple of dates and they have a lot of those characteristics that we do find desirable, then maybe it's worth committing ourselves to see where it could lead. As I said before, this is a simple commitment – nothing long term or too serious – and all that is required is the investment of some time. And if we've done our homework, we will more than likely enjoy that time because when two people are compatible, then their first few dates are usually pretty fun. Now, there is a fifty-fifty chance of "a couple of dates" turning into a special (and maybe long-term) relationship. And I've found that when you're gambling with love, fifty-fifty odds are some of the best ones a betting man can hope to find.

Now the second kind of commitment comes later in the relationship (obviously). Once a person has taken the initiative to decide that this individual deserves some of their time in order to see if they are "The One" —
...and in my case "The Two" and "The Three"...
– there then must be a decision to commit to seeing if the experiment that is now in place can work! And this is where it starts to get a little on the serious side. We are now beginning to find ourselves heading toward an agreement (commitment) to be exclusive. Now, I've never had a problem committing myself to just one woman (at a time, that is); but for some people, that can be a very scary step.

It appears to me, that most socialites possess an instinctive hesitation towards the idea of placing a limit on the number of options to which they can seek affection. But I don't think that this is the result of a fear of monogamy, I think it has more to do with a fear of failure. The idea of "making a bad choice" or "things not working out" is more than enough cause for concern when it comes to forsaking all other options and gambling on just the one choice. But that is exactly what it is – a gamble, a risk – and for me, therein lies the beauty of it all because we take risks everyday on things that are much less significant. Therefore, I have always been willing to take the gamble of committing to the chance for love because although the risks are high; the payoff is even greater.

Now this same type of commitment continues to another level, because once we take the risk of committing to a particular person, we in turn are committing to the relationship as well. And although this level of commitment is also fairly serious, it is not that complex of an issue to deal with. What I've learned from pretty much all of my marriages is that there must be an understanding between both parties that each person is committed to the institution of the relationship, and the rollercoaster ride that it will entail. For instance, the first time that we get into an argument should not mean that all bets are off. Fights and arguments are **supposed** to be a part of the relationship...they are not the checkered flag that signifies that the race is over. In fact, I devoutly believe that arguments are healthy because they reinforce the fact that we are still different from one another and have our own ideas and identities. But once the fight is over, we find a compromise on common ground (or agree to disagree) and we continue to move the relationship forward. *Also, this is the point where good make-up sex comes into*

play!
But this type of commitment takes two...it cannot be done alone. This type of commitment is where we have to put in the work because relationships are like jobs...you have to put in the time to bring home the paycheck. And if we are actually in a marriage,
-which I usually am-
then we don't even get vacations from this job because we are considered full-time employees…and that's twenty-four hours a day, seven days a week, and three hundred sixty-five days a year.
However, it does come with exceptional benefits - a loving family, a nice home, etc…

But my point is that we have to commit to contributing something everyday to our relationship because if we don't put anything in, we won't get anything out! It's simple math. And as I said before, this endeavor requires an equal commitment from both parties; it can never be just one. I can tell you from experience that if a person is committing 100% to the relationship and their partner is putting in twenty-five percent, the numbers don't equate to a successful union. Hear comes my story.

I bet you thought I was going to forget the story!

In my first marriage, I was eighteen years old and had no clue of what it took to be married; and I committed to absolutely nothing! But, my wife was twenty-one years old (and thereby more mature), and she was committed to the ground that I walked on! So while I went out and partied to the wee hours of the morning, she sat there waiting patiently for me to come home. Five plus two does not equal ten! With no clue about what was required in a marriage, I did not give anywhere near the commitment required to make it work; and as you've figured out by now, it didn't. Now on the other end of the spectrum, my third marriage was staged on more of an even playing field. And although **it** did not work out as planned either, I can honestly say that it was the one marriage that did not end due to a lack of commitment. I actually applaud her because she taught me what it meant to fight for what was important. Every time I wanted to run away at the first sign of trouble, she challenged me to stay and work through the "not so pleasant times"! And if it weren't for the fact that we just were not meant to be together, I think that this was a relationship that fundamentally could have lasted! She knew (and I learned) that the word "commitment" was not a punch line, but a real foundation of any serious relationship. Each and every day that we wake up with the person that we're committed to, we should ask ourselves, "What can I do to bring this person some happiness...what can I do to improve the quality of their life?"; and then make the effort to execute our answers. I have come to understand that this is the type of commitment that can bring joy to both sides of the romantic equator.

So as you can see, I've spent a good deal of time considering the sentiment of commitment, and how it plays a big role in our relationships. And while I've shared my thoughts with you on how I feel that there are different types of commitment, I have left for the conclusion of this chapter my belief that there are only <u>two</u> levels of any type - committed or not committed! To put it simply; we should be committed to the person that we are with and we should be committed to what we have with them. And if this is not the case, we should respect their time, as well as our own, enough to not waste it by just going through the motions.

IX: Finances

I know you're probably wondering how the topic of finances got in here when everything else that we've previously discussed has had to do with the more emotional issues, such as love and romance. Well please allow me to promptly point out (in case you have never heard this before) that bad financial interactions between two people will devastate a relationship just as quickly as anything else that we've talked about thus far. I've discovered that most of us become accustomed with dealing with our own finances our own way during the time that we are single; and then once it becomes necessary to merge our monetary lifestyle with someone of the opposite sex, things can sometimes become "sticky". And for some reason, when people are in the beginning stages of committing themselves to one another, they rarely deem it necessary to talk about this subject and it ends up being one of those issues that we determine can be "worked out" as the relationship progresses to more serious levels. But I can tell you first hand, that having a solid financial arrangement with one's significant other from the very beginning will go a long way in contributing towards the overall success (and longevity) of any union. Now in the beginning stages of my career as a professional husband, I always thought of myself as being pretty good with money; so therefore, there was never really anything that I needed to discuss with anyone else – I would handle it! But think with me back to my first chapter about "self-understanding". Remember me telling you about when I began going through my self-evaluations,

and subsequently had to realize quite a few of my shortcomings? Well, let's just say that if I were on trial for my previous financial management abilities, I would not want any of my exes to take the stand as character witnesses. In my self indulgence as a financial guru in those days, I remember having been more than inadequate at handling the "household finances" with quite a number of my fair ladies. But time waits for no man; and in an effort to catch up to it, I have learned quite a few lessons from my mistakes.
No - really I have!
It is from these lessons that I am able to offer you some of my experiences and opinions about how the handling of money (or the lack thereof) will always play an important role in any long-term relationship.

There are essentially two things I've come to understand when it comes to dealing with the joint finances of an intimate couple. The first is that there must be a mutual agreement about how money will be maintained between the two persons. As I said earlier, both parties typically come into a partnership accustomed to dealing with their own monetary affairs. And since those particular circumstances only required a singular effort, the idea of having to discuss the transactions of money with another party is one that is out of the ordinary for most individuals. A prime example of why this is important comes from my first marriage. As a new husband and wife, she and I were naturally both giddy about the idea of having a joint checking account where both of us would keep – and both have access to – all of our money. Well that immediately became a problem in our economic balance due to the fact that I had the checkbook and she had the bankcard and we were in no way communicating with one another regularly about the transactions that were being made. Needless to say, there came a point where our checks started having rubbery characteristics and phone calls started to come in from vendors who, for some reason, were upset with us. On top of that, she and I spent an enormous amount of time arguing to no end because each of us was blaming the other for who spent what money and shouldn't have. But now that I look back on those early days, I realize that this wasn't really anybody's fault; it was just the result of two young people in love who were completely inexperienced in handling money as part of a collective unit and had not had the foresight to prepare for this task early on. So through the years (and the relationships), I've come to find that the system that works best for me is one where my mate and I each have our own individual accounts that we maintain independently; and from those accounts we can both make the necessary contributions to a joint account that is used strictly for the payment of joint bills and/or purchases. It even helps to have a set day of the month where those monies need to be available so that each individual has the ability to establish a scheduled budget. That way, we can have the opportunity to predetermine together what needs to go in and come out of the joint account beforehand, while at the same time retaining the ability to still have a certain degree of control over our own monies to expedite according to our personal wants and needs. Now keep in mind that all I am saying is that this is the system that I've found to work for <u>me</u>. In no way am I suggesting that everyone should use this arrangement because every couple has a different set of circumstances that may require any one of a number of different approaches. Just because **I** wasn't able to accomplish it, doesn't mean that there aren't some couples who are very efficient in managing a collective pool of money; while there are still others who are capable of managing their finances from a single income. So, I cannot suggest that my arrangement of preference is an end all for everyone... but, what I **am** suggesting is that there should be an arrangement.

Remember, people can be very sensitive when it comes to money. And if my system does not happen to be the current situation in your home, the last thing that I want anyone to do is run out and tell their significant other that the guy who wrote that fabulous book about being a professional husband said that the two of you have to get separate bank accounts – and somebody ends up sleeping on the couch.

The point is to be sure that there is a financial structure in place that both parties are comfortable with and can adhere to. And because money can be such a touchy subject for most people, we need to ensure that whatever the plan is, it is well thought out and that it accommodates the needs of everyone involved. It has taken me many years to learn that this can save a lot of headaches and maybe even a few dollars.

The second little factoid that I picked up about love and money is that there needs to be a realistic concurrence about how financial obligations will be dispersed, and then who is going to expedite them. This seems like it wouldn't have required a lot of thought or effort on my part until the one day when the following conversation occurred:

"Honey, did you pay the light bill?" she asks me.

And my response is, "No...I thought you did."

And wouldn't you know it, this conversation happens to takes place just moments after the house had turned pitch black and the only thing visible are teeth and eyeballs. Of course, at this point there is nothing else for either of us to do in this situation but to try to play it off by pretending that we are lighting candles in preparation for a romantic dinner.

...which was hard to pull off because we had an electric stove! Please don't laugh – this actually happened to me.
All of a sudden it becomes obvious that the "we'll – work – out – the – money – as – we - go" approach to meeting our financial responsibilities probably was not the best choice we could have made after all. As I mentioned before, I feel that there are actually two things that need to be considered when it comes to monetary bliss, and the first of them is <u>how</u> the financial obligations will be distributed. I've had to use different scenarios depending on the person that I was with, but it has always come down to choosing one of a few sensible approaches. The first option, which I was only able to accomplish in my second marriage, is the most simple. It is when one of the two persons can handle all of the expenses alone, at which point the need to assign fiscal responsibilities becomes obsolete. The second scenario is also fairly basic as well, and it is the arrangement where we split the expenses fifty-fifty. So at the end of the month we sit down and compute all of the expenses for which we are jointly responsible, and exactly half of that becomes our individual obligation. Now I have found that unless both parties have fairly similar incomes, this specific scenario has a tendency to cause somewhat of a strain on the arrangement; and usually for one person in particular. When that is the case, my next option tends to be a little more accommodating. This one is when both parties share the monthly debt in proportion to individual income. In this instance, we still total up all of the joint bills at the end of the month, but we then divide the responsibility for them according to the ratio of our monthly pay. So, if I make seventy percent of the total income, then I pay seventy percent of the total bills. And vice- versa.

In all honesty, this one has proven to work the best for me, because it's fair and seems to cause almost no confrontations. And I like that!

The final method that I've tried is to assign the specific bills between both parties. Therefore, if I agree to pay the rent/mortgage, then she concurs to paying the telephone, electric, cable, etc. Now I must say that, for the most part, this scenario works well with one caveat; if something should happen to get turned off, then there is room for blame of an individual person. But hey, all of these methods have worked for me at some point and time; and as I said earlier, it was just a matter of choosing the one that was most suitable depending on the woman I was with. And I share all of this with you not as an egotistical attempt to give a lecture on Household Finance 101, but to make the point that just having a mutual understanding about how we are going to handle our finances can make life so much easier for both the king and the queen.

    Now, there is a second part to this, though, and that is determining **who** will handle the financial allocations. In my first marriage, my wife would just give me her paycheck and I was supposed to pay the bills and let her know what was left over. The only problem with that arrangement was that back in my rookie days, I had a tendency to take us out to fancy dinners or go partying with <u>bill</u> money, figuring that I could replace it or double up on something next month…which didn't always happen.
Hey, I was only eighteen years old…give me a break!
But by the time I was a veteran husband in my third marriage, I had realized that I didn't necessarily have to be the one to handle the expenses. My third wife was as competent with money as they came, and I didn't have any

question that she was capable of handling our household finances far better than I was.

Come to think of it, I don't remember anything ever getting turned off.

Anyway, I would just let her tell me how much she needed from me when I got paid and put whatever the amount was in that joint bank account I was talking about earlier. Actually, I kind of enjoyed not having the task of calculating and writing out light bills and phone bills and such; and if there was the chance that she was getting over on me…oh well, it's too late now.

My point –

Yes, I do have a point…

– is that I believe every couple needs to truthfully and realistically decide which of the two is the better economist in the relationship, and let that person handle the necessary financial obligations. And if both people are equally capable – or incapable – then maybe there can be an arrangement to share the responsibility. But, I think that once there is an understanding of **how** to handle the money and **who** will handle the money, then a humungous step has been taken to prevent an excessive amount of altercations that can arise from poor financial management. You know, they say that money makes the world go around…I say that handling it properly makes relationships last.

X: Final Thoughts

Well, here we are! I am about finished jabbering about my thoughts on what I consider to be the more important aspects of relationships; and, you now know a little about the guy who calls himself "the professional husband". In all of the previous chapters, we've talked about everything from romance to finance, and I still have not shared with you everything that flows through my mind when I think about the union between a man and a woman. But for me, if you have gotten anything out of the few romantic downfalls I have shared with you that could help make your relationship just a little bit better, then I will have accomplished what I set out to do when I began writing this book. Keep in mind, though, I have never tried to give the impression that I was giving advice or instructions; nor have I tried to pass myself off as a psychological expert on everything it takes to make a relationship work. I have simply attempted to share with you the experiences that I have endured from being married and engaged – at young ages – more times than most people do in their whole lives.

Unless you're Elizabeth Taylor, Donald Trump, or somebody like that.

But through all of the stories and all of the opinions that you've just spent a significant amount of your valuable time reading, there is one final thought that I want to leave you with. It is the one thought that I feel is the thread that connects every other subject that I've shared with you in these scribblings; and it is the paramount truth that has taken me over thirty years to discover and will probably take me thirty more to fully comprehend.

As human beings, we have an undying internal instinct that commits us to finding that one special individual who can make our lives complete – that "picture-perfect" person who satisfies the yearning in our souls. The image of that person can range anywhere from tall, dark, and handsome to short, petite, and wholesome. Over the course of our pre-adult lives and into the endeavor of our actual adulthood, we will engage in any number of relationships in search of that perfect counterpart with whom we can find happiness, bear children, and grow old. But one of the problems that I've run into trying to accomplish this seemingly simple, yet massive feat is that I hadn't set out on the correct mission. As I just stated, I was looking for that "picture-perfect" person and I spent an immoderate amount of time trying to seek her out in order to fulfill my destiny. But after many travels and much heartbreak, I have been brought to an ultimate realization that has shaken the very core of my being. I've come to believe that there is **no** such thing. There is no "perfect" spouse, no "perfect" relationship, or no "perfect" marriage. But. There are imperfect people who can have a perfect commitment to working on a still imperfect relationship so that it has a perfect ending for them. Let me explain.

"Nobody is perfect." That is a cliché that we have all used to justify some shortcoming that someone else has taken the time to point out in us. However, whenever we are not the actual person saying these words, we tend to forget this ageless fact when it comes to the individual with whom we might be finding fault. So I've tried to take it from the perspective of having an even playing field when it comes to relationships. For as much as I may think she's screwed up, she almost certainly will feel the same way about me…and typically we'll both be right. But in this situation, loving each other should give us the ability to accept one another; not only for those wonderful attributes that have drawn us together in the first place, but also for the flaws that connect us as human beings. I think that a perfect relationship is one where we are able and willing to accept the faults in our partner and they are able and willing to do the same for us. And not only do we accept them, but we do everything within our power to cover up their shortcomings, and they reciprocate this act for us. It's what I call a perfect fit – when any negative (meaning shortcoming or fault) about our character is complimented by a positive trait in the persona of our partner. And I believe that when this type of interaction exists in a relationship, the chances of lifetime unity increases by the odds of infinity. Now at this juncture, I do want to go back and reiterate a point I made earlier in the book –

I think it was the chapter on Commitment. You would think I would know since I am the one doing the writing, huh?

Being able to accept the faults of another person is contingent upon identifying those faults and making the actual decision to accept them early in the relationship. For instance, if two people meet and one person is a smoker and the other is not, then the non-smoker should decide up front whether or not this is a trait that they are willing to accept in the person that they have fallen for. It should not be something that, in the back of their mind, the non-smoker feels that they will be able to change about the other person over time. I am a deep advocate of the idea that change in people comes from within, not from the external influence of others. And I have learned from many experiences that we cannot change our counterparts to become the person that we want them to be. Attempting to do this has proven to produce either one – or both – of two results. The first is that a person will make the effort to change, but it is only temporary and they will eventually revert back to their original (and natural) form. The second result is that the individual will make the effort to change, but they will ultimately come to resent the one who forced this change upon them. Both of these scenarios are counterproductive to a relationship and have both claimed responsibility for quite a few heartbreaks in the life of the professional husband. And the lesson I've learned: Either accept someone for who they are or don't accept them at all!

Now I'm spending my closing moments with you talking about faults and imperfections because these topics are subplots to the grander theme in my final thought. If you'll remember a few paragraphs ago, I made the statement "There is no "perfect" spouse, no "perfect" relationship, or no "perfect" marriage…" Well, I believe this immensely and I think that we as humans spend way too much time concentrating on the "little things" when it comes to love. Far too many times, I have spent an inordinate amount of energy focusing on the minor characteristics in my mate that didn't necessarily please me; as opposed to relishing the more dominant, positive traits she had to offer that actually made me happy.

"She's too tall" or "her hair's too short" or "she doesn't like sports the way that I do"…you'd be amazed at some of the things that have made me decide that any given relationship was not going to work out!

But as I've matured over the years, I have learned that a majority of the time, most of these things are irrelevant in the grand scheme of things. I've come to understand that concentrating my romantic efforts on the more significant qualities of my intimate counterpart is essential to being able to maintain a substantial and wholesome relationship. I can think of quite a few women who would have made any sacrifice or engaged in any legal (and sometimes, illegal) activity just to make me happy. And for some reason, that type of commitment and loyalty was not enough for me. Maybe she was a little sassier than I would have liked, or she didn't clean house the way that I wanted it cleaned; therefore I chose to overlook the sincere devotion that this person was exhibiting towards me every single day. I was searching for perfection – a fairy tale – and nothing else would do! But you know what? I've had to change <u>what</u> I was looking for and <u>where</u> I was looking for it.

I finally came to the conclusion that the "fairy tale" that I have been chasing all this time was **not** to be found somewhere between here and the furthest outposts of our planet; it only exists within the confines of my heart! I have discovered that love between two people is not the result of any supernatural force that has some type of external influence over their destinies, but it is the product of an unadulterated, emotional commitment that each individual has decided to entrust to the other. Believe me, I've tried every approach known to civilized man; and I've come to the astoundingly simplistic realization that true love is what we make it. It has finally dawned on me that when another person is able and willing to match the love and commitment in an equal proportion of which I am investing in the relationship, then that is the **beginning** of my fairy tale…not the ending. It's funny; for all of this time I have been so caught up in the miniscule complexities of what my ideal person should be like, I didn't take the opportunity to search for the most basic of my necessities. I've come to terms with the idea that when we lie in our beds at night and look at the person across from us, there are two questions that we should ask ourselves.

"Do I truly love this person and do they truly love me?"

"Do I think this person will do everything they can to protect my well-being and am I prepared to do the same for them?"

I know they are both two-part questions, which really makes if four, but indulge me on the technicality.

I sincerely believe that if you can answer "yes" without a shadow of a doubt to both of these questions, then everything else is insignificant. I mean, when it really comes down to what's important, aren't these the only two things that are non-negotiable when it comes to who we want to spend our lives with. When these emotions are a certainty, does anything else – like whether a person is too short or too tall, or not funny enough or too serious – does any of that really matter? My numerous encounters with love have brought me to the belief that it doesn't. And this is the idea that brings me to the point that I've been trying to make – my final thought. Love the someone who loves you…take care of the someone who takes care of you; and in doing so, be willing to accept everything else in between!

Oh, Lord. Please give me the courage to change the things that I can, the serenity to accept the things I cannot change; and the wisdom to know the difference!

Finally, I pray that no one within the grasp of my words will ever acquire the marital experience that is necessary to obtain the title of a "professional husband (or wife)". It is my hope that each of you will find the one person with whom you can share the "fairy tale" within your heart. And as I leave you now, I will attempt to humor you with a rendition of one of my favorite commercials:

The cost of love: A little vulnerability.

The cost of communication: A little effort.

The cost of togetherness: A little time.

The cost of a lifetime of joy and happiness with the one you love:

Priceless!

Afterword

I would like to take one last minute of your time before you go to clarify two particular points that I felt were hindsight as I completed this book.

First, when I began writing this short story, I was in fact engaged to Fiancé #3. However; during the time it took me to complete my writings, Fiancé #3 became Wife #4. And I felt it pertinent to mention this because it was during the complications that led to the end of that marriage that I received the inspiration to finally complete this book. So in fact, there were ultimately <u>four</u> wives and two fiancés from whom I drew the experiences on which my stories are based.

Now, the reason for yet a Third Edition of this book is that from the time I completed and published the first two editions, I have since married for a FIFTH time! I know your eyes probably just popped open to the size of two golf balls and your head is shaking in disbelief, but if you'll remember back to the beginning chapters, I affirmed that I was hopelessly willing to "jump the broom" again! And the fact that Marriage #5 did not turn out as I had hoped has made me more determined than ever to share my story in the hope that my experiences will in fact help someone somewhere avoid mistakes in any way similar to the ones I've faced!

My second point is that my reference to myself as "the professional husband" is purely for a comical effect. It began when (prior to starting this book) I once visited my family with (then) Fiancé #3 back when we had just started dating. My siblings and cousins were teasing me about the number of times I had been married and the fact that it appeared that I was at it again. In an effort to mask my embarrassment and self-disappointment at the truth of their remarks, I made my own joke of the situation by replying that I would do it as many times as it took because I was a professional husband. And so the playful legend began. I wanted to be sure that you knew this story because in no way do I want anyone to think that I take the institution of marriage lightly and that I do not respect it. I do, and probably more than I can ever express. I have only used this lighthearted reference to a professional husband as a vehicle through which I could grab the attention of my audience to be able to share my story. It is my deepest desire that every person who has taken the time to read my book either has already found, or will in the near future find, that one special person with whom they can have that "forever" type relationship.

I sincerely thank you for your time and patronage!

And I wish you a life of love with the love of your life!

-Broderick X. Thomas, Sr.-

About The Author

Broderick Thomas was born and raised in the small town of South Hill, VA. After graduating high school, he enlisted in the United States Air Force for a four-year tour. Upon leaving the military, he spent several more years in the city of his last duty station, Denver, CO, before moving back to his home state of Virginia. Broderick now resides in Richmond, VA, where he has spent the last 17 years in marketing and advertising. He has one child, Broderick Xavier, Jr. and a grandson, Dominic Xavier. His passions are reading, sports activities (particularly coaching little league football) and serving in ministry. Broderick spent three years as a student at ***Spirit of Faith Bible Institute*** in Maryland where he graduated with a Diploma of Ministerial Studies in June 2011.

Email The Professional Husband at:

broderick@theprofessionalhusband.com